Fast Facts for Patients

AF848669

Oncology
—
Pneumology

# First, the facts...

1. Non-small cell lung cancer (NSCLC) is one of two main types of lung cancer.
2. Some lung cancers spread to other parts of the body before they are diagnosed. A cancer that has spread is called 'metastatic'.
3. New lung cancer treatments are being developed that directly target the gene mutations that control how cancers grow and spread.
4. The most important gene mutations in cancer are called 'driver mutations'. In NSCLC, this includes KRAS mutations, which can be used as targets for treatment.
5. There are new treatments designed for lung cancers with a KRAS mutation that are already available. And more are being developed.
6. Treatments in development are tested in clinical trials. There are several different phases of clinical trials that people with cancer can take part in.

**This booklet aims to help you understand your options so you can talk to your doctors, nurses, and medical team about your cancer and its treatment. Use the spaces on the pages to organize your notes and questions.**

Karger

HEALTHCARE

## What is non-small cell lung cancer?

Non-small cell lung cancer – abbreviated to NSCLC – is one of the two main types of lung cancer; 85% of lung cancers are NSCLC, the other 15% are called small cell lung cancers.

There are three main types of NSCLC that develop from different types of lung cells.

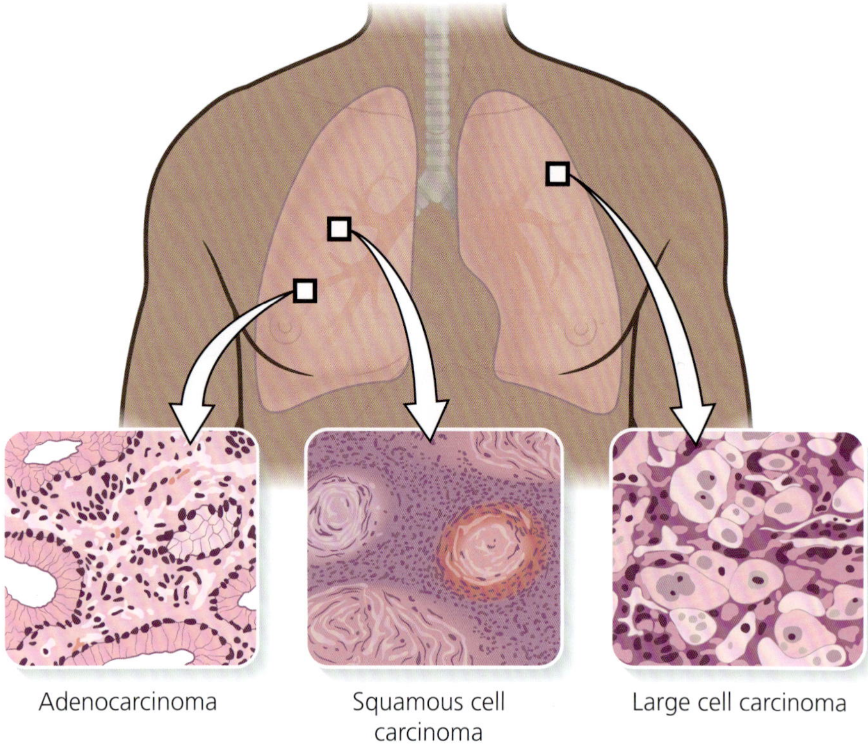


**Adenocarcinoma** develops from gland cells in the lungs, which produce mucus. The mucus helps to trap any irritants that get into your airways so you can get rid of them by coughing. Around 4 in 10 lung cancers (40%) are this type.

**Squamous cell carcinoma** develops from flat cells that line the inside of the airways of the lungs. Around 3 in 10 lung cancers (30%) are this type.

**Large cell carcinoma** usually develops in the outer area of the lungs. It's called that because the cancer cells look particularly large under a microscope. These cancers are sometimes called 'undifferentiated'. That means the cells are not specialized as normal lung cells are. About 1 in 10 lung cancers (10%) are this type.

There are other subtypes of NSCLC that are much rarer. Together, they make up about 1 in 20 cases (5%).

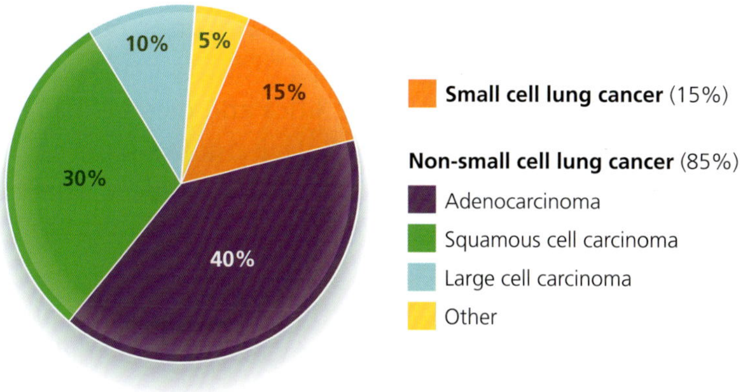


**Questions for your doctor**

*Make a note of any questions you may have...*

## How can lung cancer develop?

We can't tell exactly what causes each case of lung cancer. But there are risk factors we do know about.

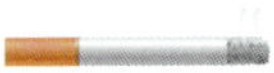

Tobacco smoke is the main risk factor for lung cancer, causing about 8 out of 10 cases (80%).

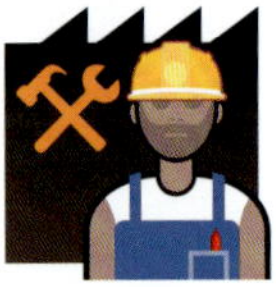

Some people get lung cancer because of substances they've been exposed to. Asbestos – a fibre used for insulation – is a severe lung irritant that can cause cancer many years later. It's now banned in many countries, but people working in the building industry may come into contact with it. Silica and diesel exhaust fumes are other workplace risk factors.

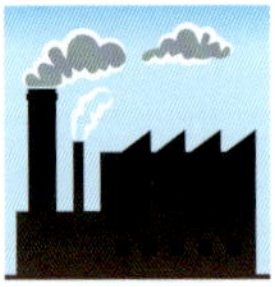

Air pollution can cause lung cancer. The risk varies, depending on the levels of pollution where you live and work.

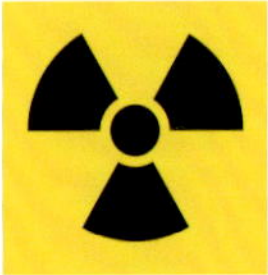

There is radiation that occurs naturally in rocks, water, and air, as well as cosmic radiation that comes from space. Radon gas is produced by the natural decay of uranium. Levels are higher in some areas than others and can increase the risk of lung cancer, particularly for people with a history of smoking.

### Why do some people get cancer and not others?

Everyone is at risk of developing lung cancer, irrespective of their smoking history. However, smoking can interact with other factors and increase your risk. Some people are more prone to cancer than others, particularly if there are other cases in their close family.

Some cancers occur randomly, and we never know the cause. And some may be due to risk factors we don't know about yet.

## What is metastatic NSCLC?

Metastatic cancer (also known as 'advanced cancer') means that a cancer has spread from where it first started in the body. A metastatic lung cancer is one that has spread from the lung to another body organ. The cancer cells do this by breaking away from the tumor and traveling through the bloodstream or the lymphatic system. The cells settle somewhere else and start to grow into new tumors.

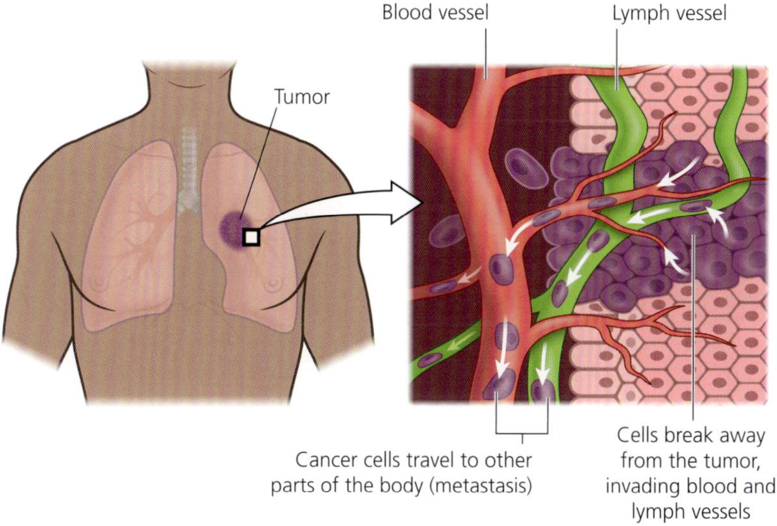


### Primary and secondary cancer

Where the cancer starts is called the primary cancer. Where the cancer spreads to is called a secondary cancer.

NSCLC can spread to several places, such as the bones, liver, and brain. Because the cells that have spread are lung cancer cells, it's still a lung cancer, not a liver or bone cancer. It's important to understand this. Because these secondary cancers are made of lung cancer cells, they will respond best to treatment that has been proven to treat lung cancer, not primary liver cancer or primary bone cancer.

Sometimes cancers aren't found until they've already spread. A primary cancer may be small and cause few or no symptoms. But if cells have broken away from the main tumor and started to grow elsewhere, these secondary cancers may cause symptoms that lead to diagnosis.

**Commonly used words**

There are lots of different terms that doctors use about cancer, and it helps to know what they mean.

The **primary** cancer site is where the cancer first started growing in the body. With NSCLC, the primary cancer site is the lung.

A **secondary** cancer site is where a primary cancer has spread to. It's the same type of cancer as the primary cancer, just growing somewhere else in the body.

**Metastatic** cancer (sometimes called **mets**) means a cancer that has spread to another part of the body.

You may hear your doctor talk about **staging**. This is how doctors describe how far a cancer has grown and whether it has spread. There are usually four main **cancer stages**. A small, localized cancer is stage 1. A stage 4 cancer means the same as metastatic cancer – a cancer that has spread to another part of the body.

## Finding out that you have metastatic cancer

It's a shock to find out a cancer has spread. Whether it's come back after earlier treatment for a primary cancer or had already spread when you were diagnosed, it's difficult news to hear. It's also difficult news to pass on to your close friends and family.

People may tell you to 'keep positive' or even that 'being positive will help fight your cancer'. But there's no right or wrong way to feel. You don't have to keep up a cheerful front all the time. You can have a positive attitude and still feel worried or upset.

Reliable sources of support and information are important. It may help to talk to others in the same situation as you. The internet makes this easier than ever. There are also likely to be local support groups where you can meet other people affected by cancer. Ask at your cancer center. You can also ask your healthcare team about available mental health/counseling resources, care giver support, or financial planning help.

Positivity also means being hopeful. New treatments are being developed all the time. In fact, that's what this booklet is about. There are now more treatments for metastatic lung cancer than ever before. Even if it's not possible to completely get rid of your cancer, there are treatments that might control it.

Your family and friends will want to support you, even if they are worried and not sure how best to do it. Let them know what you need. Just listening to you while you talk through concerns can be a great help.

**My sources of support are...**

*My online forum(s) and support groups are at:*

*My local support group is at:*

## More about genes and cancer

Cancer treatment has been developing over the past few decades. Genes can become abnormal, enabling cancers to grow and spread; researchers are now finding ways to target these abnormal genes. To understand this type of treatment, which is often referred to as 'targeted treatment', it helps to understand a bit about how cancers start.

Everything that cells do starts with their genes, which are made of **DNA** and carry instructions for making **proteins**. Normal cells need these proteins to work properly. Proteins control how cells grow and become specialized, as well as controlling every function of each cell.

### Gene mutations and cancer

Cells can become cancerous because they have changes (**mutations**) in their genes. Some mutations are inherited from a parent, are present from birth, and can be passed on to children. Others develop during a person's lifetime and can't be passed on.

Mutations cause the affected genes to make abnormal proteins that can prevent the cell from working properly. Not all mutations result in a cancer. But some give the cell properties that make it more likely to become cancerous if it collects a few more mutations.

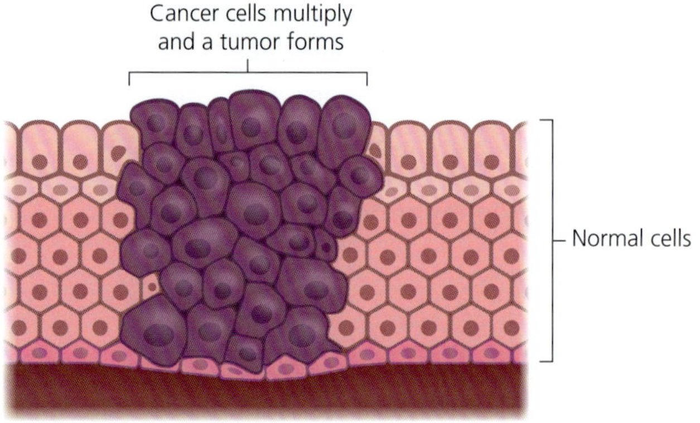

The most obvious cancer-causing mutations are those that cause the cell to keep multiplying when it shouldn't. Normally in adults, most cells only reproduce to replace worn-out cells and repair damage. But cancer cells carry on multiplying much more quickly than normal cells do. The excess cells form a lump – a tumor.

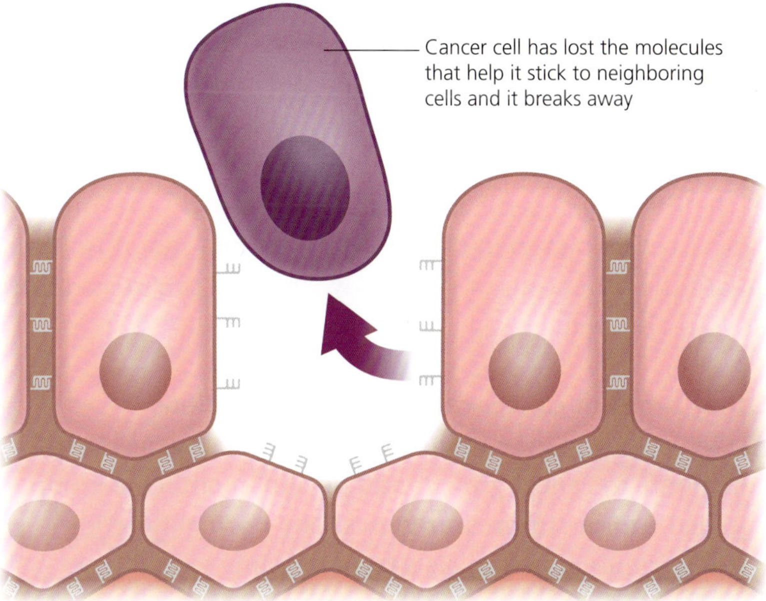


There are other mutations that mean the cells lose their ability to stick together. This is one reason why cancers are able to spread. Cancer cells can break away and travel through the blood and lymphatic system to another part of the body and start growing there. Once a cell has a mutation, it will pass it on every time it divides.

## Oncogenes and cancer

Mutated forms of genes involved in normal cell division are called **oncogenes**. They can encourage cancer growth and development.

Sometimes oncogene mutations that lead to cancer are inherited – the breast cancer genes BRCA1 and BRCA2, for instance. More commonly, mutations happen because of cancer-causing substances we're exposed to, such as ultraviolet rays from the sun or smoking tobacco. These mutations are only found in cells that have become damaged. So, if you're told your lung cancer has a mutation in the **KRAS** oncogene, this mutation is only in the lung cancer cells. You weren't born with the mutation, it isn't in any of the other cells of your body, and you can't pass it on to your children.

### Other types of cancer-causing gene mutations

As well as oncogenes, there are other types of genes that contribute to cancer growth and development. One group is called **tumor suppressor genes**. The normal function of these genes is to stop cells from dividing when they shouldn't. In many tumors, however, mutations in these genes mean they are lost or inactivated. This allows the cells to continue to divide and the cancer develops.

Other cancer-causing genes are called **DNA repair genes**. In normal cells, these genes repair damage caused to the DNA. If the DNA damage is too bad, the DNA repair gene will tell the cell to self-destruct.

Cells with mutations in these DNA repair genes are less able to repair cancer-causing mutations. They are also able to survive with DNA damage that would cause normal cells to die.

## Driver mutations

The most important gene changes in the development of cancer cells are called **driver mutations** – because they drive the development of a cancer. An abnormal protein produced because of a driver mutation may be key to encouraging cancer cells to keep on dividing, for example.

These important mutations are being researched as potential targets for treatment. If treatments can block the proteins that these genes make, they can help to stop cancer growth and might keep people healthy for longer.

## KRAS mutations are driver mutations

Normal KRAS protein is important in the control of cell replacement and development. But KRAS mutations can produce abnormal proteins that are permanently active, instead of only working when they need to. These proteins encourage cells to multiply all the time.

There are several different mutations in the KRAS gene that we know are possible driver mutations for lung cancer. Each individual cancer is likely to have only one type of driver mutation.

## Driver mutations and biomarkers

A biomarker is a characteristic of the body that can be measured. There are different types of biomarkers. For instance, a biomarker may be used to diagnose a disease, measure a normal body process, or show how a treatment is working.

If a diagnostic biomarker is present, that confirms a diagnosis. Some biomarkers are used to monitor a condition. For example, excess PSA is made by prostate cancer cells, so levels rise when a prostate cancer is growing.

**Types of question that can sometimes be answered by cancer biomarkers**

**Prognostic:** How aggressive is the cancer likely to be?

**Diagnostic:** What type of cancer is it?

**Predictive:** Is this the optimal drug for my cancer?

**Recurrence:** Will the cancer return?

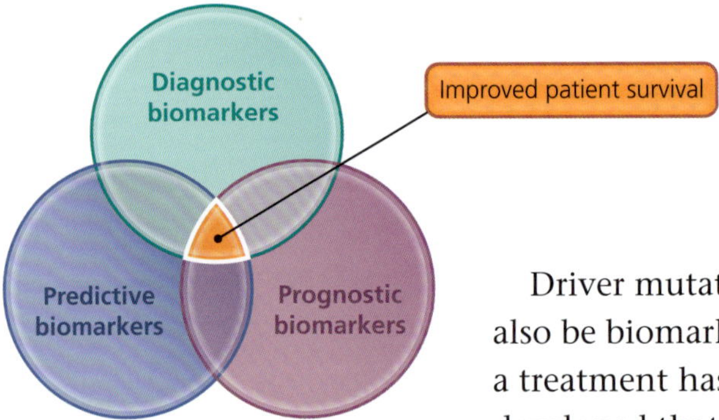


Biomarker information can be combined to improve patient survival

Driver mutations can also be biomarkers. If a treatment has been developed that targets a driver mutation, the presence of the abnormal protein produced as a result of the mutation in your cancer cells shows your doctor that this type of treatment could work for you. But not all cancers have a specific driver mutation.

## Biomarkers in lung cancer

There are several different biomarkers in lung cancer. The most common include **EGFR**, **ALK**, and **KRAS**.

**EGFR** is a gene that normally encourages cells to divide. But if mutated, it causes too much cell division, which can result in a cancer. There are several different EGFR mutations that can lead to lung cancer. Some of these can be targets for treatments called EGFR inhibitors.

**ALK** is a gene that normally helps in the development of the gut and nervous system, and is switched off after this is completed in the womb. Sometimes ALK gets switched back on again, fuses with another gene, and causes lung cancer. Treatments that target ALK are called ALK inhibitors.

**KRAS** is the biomarker that we're most interested in here. You've been given this booklet because your lung cancer has tested positive for a specific KRAS mutation and might respond to treatment that blocks the abnormal protein made by it.

**Questions for your doctor**

*Make a note of any questions you may have...*

## How your doctor knows your cancer is KRAS-positive

To find out if your cancer is KRAS-positive, your doctor took a sample of cancer cells for testing (a biopsy). You may have had this done when you were first diagnosed, through a **bronchoscopy** or a **needle biopsy**. Or the cells may have been tested when you had surgery to remove your primary cancer.

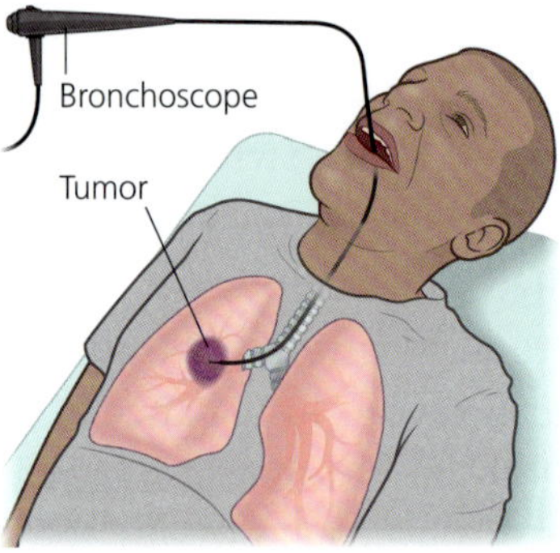


Bronchoscopy

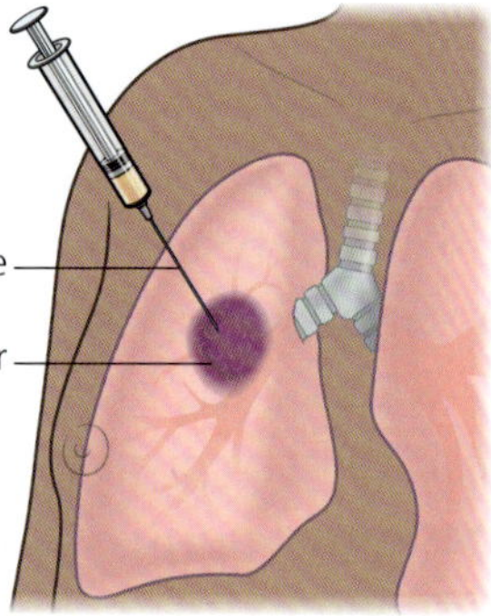


Needle biopsy

Mutations can change in cancers as they grow, so your doctor may have re-tested your cancer cells. You may have had a blood test to do this, as genetic material from the cancer can in some cases be detected in blood samples. Your doctor may call this a '**liquid biopsy**'. Or you may have had a sample of secondary cancer taken, for example through a **liver biopsy** or a **lymph-node biopsy**.

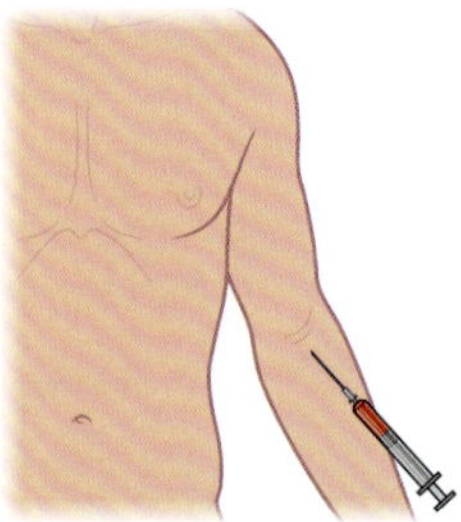

Liquid biopsy

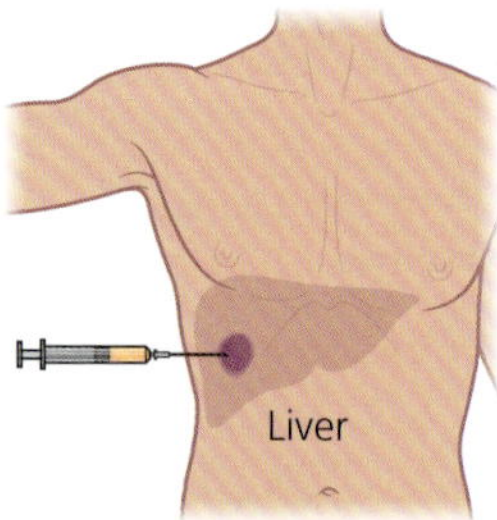


Liver biopsy

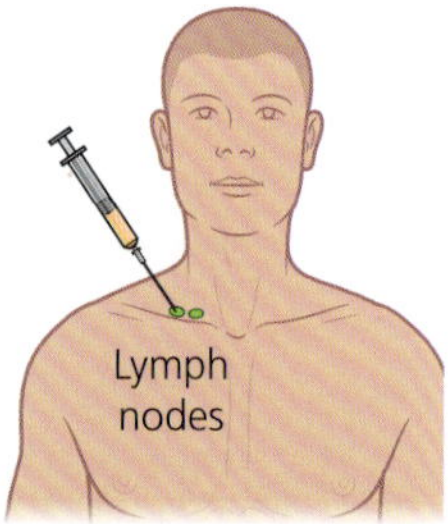


Lymph-node biopsy

## More about KRAS

KRAS and its importance in the development of cancers was discovered over 30 years ago. It was first found in human cancer cells in the early 1980s. Soon, scientists had identified KRAS mutations in a whole range of cancers and realized its importance. They now calculate that some type of KRAS mutation is found in more than 1 in 5 (20%) of all cancers. Around 1 in 4 (25%) NSCLCs have KRAS mutations.

KRAS is associated with some cancer types more than others. KRAS mutations are nearly always found in adenocarcinomas (cancers that develop from gland cells in the lung). They are also more common in:

- people who are or were tobacco smokers
- people who were exposed to asbestos in the past
- some ethnic groups compared with others: for example, they are found in up to 1 in 2 (50%) lung cancers diagnosed in White populations compared with 1 in 6 (around 17%) diagnosed in populations with lung cancer from Asia.

### KRAS subtypes in NSCLC

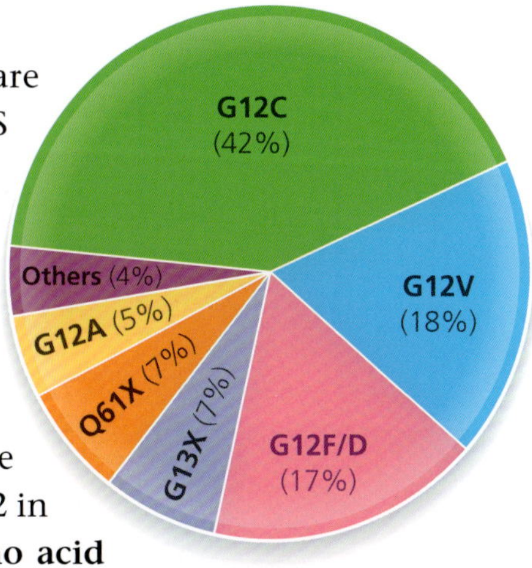


We now know that there are different types of KRAS mutations. These are named after the point in the gene where the mutation occurs and the change that takes place. As you can see, the G12C mutation is much more common than the others. The mutation occurs at position 12 in the KRAS gene and the **amino acid** C (cysteine) is substituted for the G (glycine) amino acid. Amino acids link together to form proteins.

Treatments are being developed by several pharmaceutical companies that specifically target this mutation. Other treatments are being developed that hopefully will work for several types of KRAS mutation. Ask your specialist what type of mutations they've found in your lung cancer cells. It'll help you to understand which treatments may help.

**Questions for your doctor on lung cancer mutation(s)**

*Have any mutations been found in my lung cancer cells?*

*What are the implications of the mutation(s) for my lung cancer?*

*Is there any treatment that targets the lung cancer mutation(s) I have?*

## What does having a KRAS-positive cancer mean for me?

If you have an NSCLC that has a KRAS mutation, this information will tell your doctor which treatment option is likely to work best for you. This section tells you more about KRAS-**targeted treatment** and other treatment options that are in development for KRAS-positive NSCLC.

### KRAS-targeted therapies

At the time of writing there are two KRAS-targeted therapies that are approved for treating NSCLCs with a G12C KRAS mutation. These therapies are sotorasib and adagrasib. To have this treatment, you must have:

- an NSCLC with the G12C KRAS mutation
- cancer that has spread from the lung into nearby body tissues or to somewhere else in the body
- already tried at least one other type of '**systemic**' treatment for your cancer spread (such as chemotherapy or immunotherapy).

Treatments that target other less-common types of KRAS mutations are also being researched. There are also 'universal' KRAS-targeted therapies in development. These may work across several different types of KRAS mutation. If you don't have a G12C mutation in your lung cancer cells, your doctor may suggest having one of these treatments as part of a **clinical trial**.

### How KRAS-targeted treatment works

To understand how this type of treatment works, it may help to think of it as a switch that turns off the cancer's ability to grow.

As we've seen, the cancer cells produce an abnormal form of the KRAS protein. This permanently switches on the cells' drive to divide and multiply, causing the cancer to grow.

KRAS-targeted treatment acts as a block on the abnormal protein. It attaches (binds) to it and stops it from delivering the message telling the cancer cells to divide.

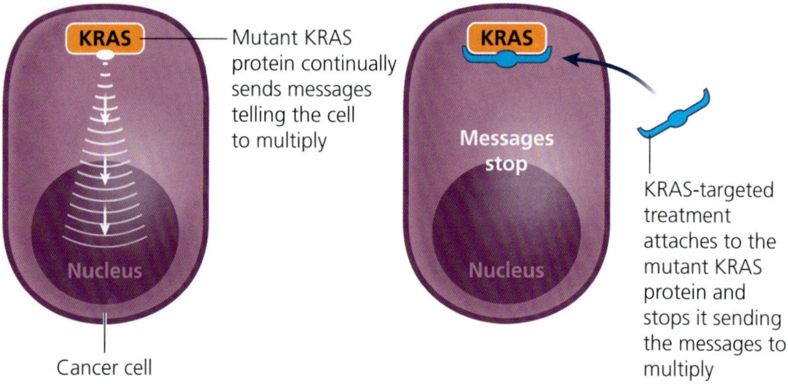


**Commonly used words**

You may hear your doctor talk about **systemic therapy**.

A systemic therapy is one that circulates through the bloodstream and treats cancer wherever it is in the body. Any treatment you take as a tablet or have through a drip (IV [intravenous] infusion) into a vein is systemic.

In cancer care, chemotherapy, hormone therapy, immunotherapy, and targeted therapies given by mouth or by injection are called 'systemic'.

Cancers that have spread are generally treated with systemic therapies because they can reach the cancer cells wherever they are in the body.

## How KRAS-targeted treatment is helping

Before treatments were developed, people with KRAS-positive advanced NSCLC didn't do as well as those without a KRAS mutation in their tumors. But KRAS-targeted treatment may change that.

Clinical trials have looked at treating advanced NSCLC with the G12C mutation. More than 1 in 3 (33%) patients who participated in the trials had their cancer shrink or stop growing for a few months. These were early Phase I and II trials. Research is ongoing in later-phase randomized trials (see the section on clinical trials on page 22 for more about trial phases).

Sadly, we know that the treatment currently available will not permanently stop advanced lung cancer from growing. In these trials, the treatment controlled advanced disease for approximately 6 to 7 months.

> **IMPORTANT:** Statistics apply to the overall population of trial participants and can't predict what will happen in your case. They can only be a general guide to what may help you. It's best to discuss this with your own specialist, who has all the test results that apply to **you**.

Trials are now looking into whether KRAS-targeted therapy may help when combined with other types of treatment, such as chemotherapy or immunotherapy.

So far, we only know that KRAS-targeting treatments can help with advanced disease. But now researchers are starting to look into whether the treatment could help people with early-stage lung cancer.

### KRAS vaccines and genetic engineering

Researchers are currently looking into creating vaccines that target KRAS mutations in people with advanced lung cancer and at modifying a patient's own immune system cells to help them target cancer cells. Both these types of treatment are still in the early stages of research.

## Talking to your doctor about your treatment

The reason a doctor suggests a new treatment for advanced cancer is often because the treatment you're on is no longer helping. This can be devastating to hear. It's common for people to focus on it so much that they don't hear anything else that's said.

It may be more helpful to talk about any new treatment options at another appointment, when you've had time to sort out what you'd like to ask.

It's a good idea to make a plan for the appointment by listing the questions you have. If you know you will be discussing something new with your doctor, it can help to take someone with you. They may pick up on things that you miss and vice versa.

Some doctors are happy for you to record consultations – but ask for permission first.

Your doctor has spent many years studying cancer care, and cancer is complicated. If you don't understand something, ask your doctor to explain in a different way. You don't have to know or use technical terms – but there is a guide to words and phrases in the back of this booklet if you want to know what they mean.

If you're not eligible for current KRAS-targeted treatment, you may be eligible to participate in a clinical trial. If you're interested, ask your doctor for more details.

**Questions for your doctor about KRAS-targeted therapy**

*If you're eligible for current KRAS-targeted therapy, questions for your doctor may include:*

*What are the aims of this treatment?*

*How do I take the treatment?*

*How many times a day do I take it?*

*Can I take the treatment at home?*

*Can I continue to take other prescribed medicines?*

*What should I do if I miss a dose?*

*What should I do if I am sick after taking a dose?*

*For how long will I take the treatment?*

*What should I do if I have difficulty swallowing it?*

*What are the most common side effects?*

*How will I be monitored when I am on the treatment?*

The next section talks about what happens in a clinical trial, things to think about if you're considering taking part, and where you can go to get more information.

## About clinical trials and research

There are different types of clinical trials, looking into screening or diagnosis for instance. The trials that are sometimes of most interest to people already diagnosed with cancer are trials that test new treatments.

### Phases of clinical trials

A new treatment must go through several phases of clinical trials to prove that it works better than existing treatment and can be adopted into routine care. A potential treatment will only move on to the next phase of research if it is safe and shows promise.

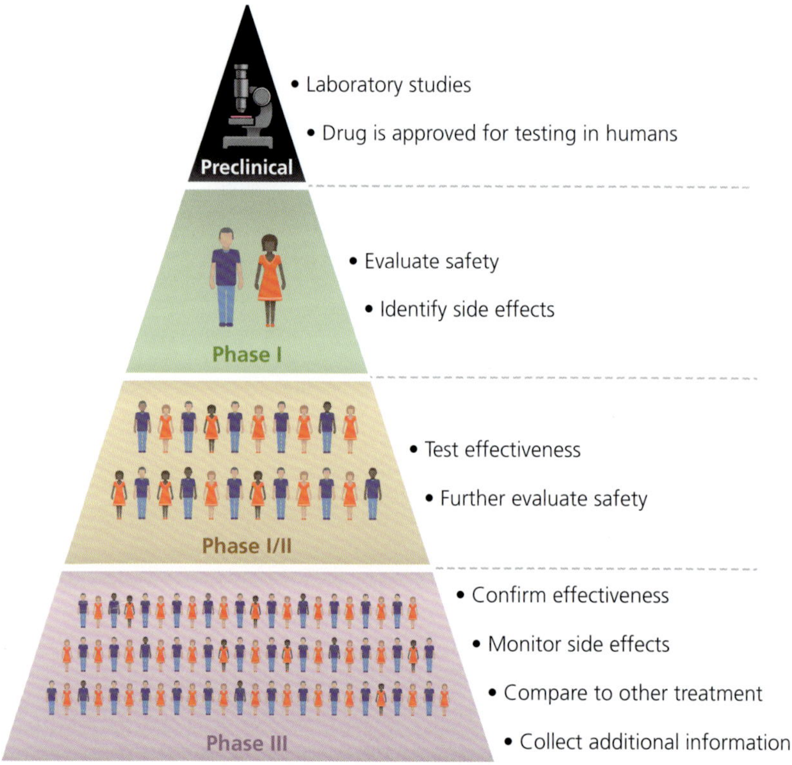

### Phase 0 and I trials

The earliest-phase trials are Phase 0 and Phase I. These are usually very small trials, involving 10–50 people. Their aim is to find out if a potential new treatment is safe, what the side effects are, and what happens to the treatment in the body (how your body gets rid of a drug, for example). Researchers may include a number of different cancer types in these early-phase trials.

### Phase II trials

Once a treatment is found to be relatively safe, a Phase II trial may take place. This is a medium-sized trial, usually of fewer than 100 people. Phase II trials usually focus on one or two cancer types that the treatment worked best for in earlier trials.

The aim of Phase II trials is to find out more about side effects and see how well a treatment works for specific types of cancer. Sometimes Phase II trials are randomized, but generally not (there is more about randomization in the section below on Phase III trials).

### Phase III trials

Phase III is the largest phase of a clinical trial and is most likely what people think of when they think about research. The aim is to test a new treatment against a treatment that is already in use to see which works better for a particular type and stage of cancer. But Phase III trials also collect more side-effect data and look at the quality of life of those having each treatment.

Usually, hundreds or even thousands of people take part in a Phase III trial, and they are often international. These trials are usually randomized. Randomized means that participants are put into two or more groups to compare the existing treatment and the new treatment. The groups have

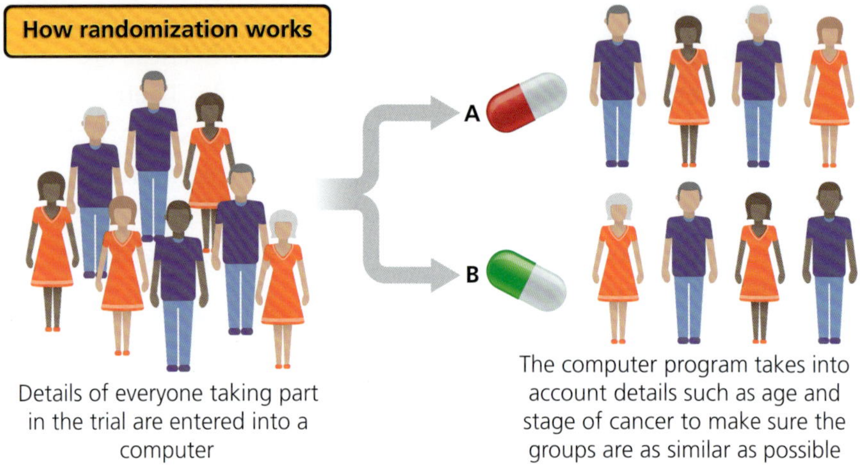


to be as similar as possible. You can't choose which group you're in, because that could affect the results.

Participants in Phase III trials are monitored by the researchers for a number of years afterwards. This is to see how well each treatment works in the long term – whether it stops an early cancer coming back or controls an advanced cancer for longer. Phase III trials often take several years to show a result.

## Phase IV trials

Phase IV trials are often referred to as 'post-marketing studies', and are conducted after a treatment is approved. These trials provide additional information on the treatment, including risks, benefits, and best use.

## The benefits and risks of taking part in a trial

A common reason people have for entering a clinical trial is that it may give them access to an experimental treatment. Many people also feel that they are giving something back and that by taking part they can help people with cancer in the future.

Remember, if you enter a randomized trial, you may or may not get the experimental treatment. You may not know which treatment you're getting, as many randomized trials are 'blinded'. Blinded means the doctors and researchers running the trial don't know who is having which treatment. This information is kept secret ('blinded') until it's time to analyze the results.

With any experimental treatment, there is no absolute guarantee of safety. Treatments are tested thoroughly before they are given to people. With each phase of research, more is learned about possible side effects. But the treatment won't have been given to large numbers of people, and not all side effects may be fully known.

As well as treatment, trials can often mean that you have more tests and scans than usual. Some people feel this is a benefit – they are having more check-ups and so feel reassured. Others find it stressful. There may be travel involved too, back and forth to the treatment center, though some costs may be covered by the organizer of the trial. It's worth thinking about the time commitment too, and the impact more tests may have on your well-being before you join a trial.

Trials often have very strict entry (**eligibility**) criteria. This is so they can make accurate comparisons between groups of participants.

**You will only be able to enter trials that are suitable for you. Suitable trials are those looking into treatment for your type and stage of cancer.** There may also be restrictions on entry for treatments you've had in the past or other medical conditions you might have.

You have to give your formal consent to take part in a trial. Before you sign, the researchers have a legal obligation to tell you about:

- the trial aims
- the treatments
- the potential benefits and risks, including side effects
- the tests and check-ups you'll need
- how long you'll have to come for follow-up appointments
- whether they will be keeping tissue or blood samples for future research.

They'll give you a **patient information sheet** to take away with you, with all of this information written down.

You don't have to decide immediately whether you'll join or not. It's important to say if you'd like some time to think it over, and maybe talk things over with those closest to you. Ask if there's a number you can call if you have further questions about participating.

Please don't feel obliged to enter a trial. If you don't, your doctor won't be offended or upset, and it won't affect your current treatment. And it's important to know that you can withdraw from (leave) a trial whenever you want. You don't have to give a reason.

### How to find out about clinical trials

The easiest way to find out about clinical trials is to ask your own specialist. They have access to all of your test results and past treatments, so they can tell you which trials are suitable for you (and which you are likely to be eligible for).

Depending on where you live, you may also be able to find clinical trials online. There are cancer clinical trials databases based in the UK, Europe, and the USA.

The US National Library of Medicine (NLM) runs a clinical trials database that has information on trials running worldwide. It isn't written for patients, so it can be difficult to understand. But you can search specifically for NSCLC trials and by country.

https://clinicaltrials.gov

The European Union Drug Regulating Authorities Clinical Trials Database is the European database for all interventional clinical trials on medicinal products taking place in the European Union/European Economic Area. Again, this isn't written for the public, so it can be difficult to read.

https://eudract.ema.europa.eu

Cancer Research UK has a clinical trials database that is written specifically for the public, in plain English. It only lists trials that are active in the UK (but of course this does include some international trials). You can search for NSCLC trials, by trial phase, and for trials in England, Scotland, Wales, or Northern Ireland.

www.cancerresearchuk.org/about-cancer/find-a-clinical-trial

### What to ask about a clinical trial

If you are considering taking part in a clinical trial, it may be helpful to think through what you'd like to know before you join.

As well as finding out about the trial aims and treatments, there are practical concerns, such as how much time you'll need to spend having tests, treatment, and check-ups. There may be hidden costs, such as parking and hotel stays. Ask if any financial support is available to help with these.

## Questions for your doctor about clinical trials

*Are there any trials I could enter that are for my type and stage of cancer?*

*What treatment can you offer if I decide not to enter a trial?*

*What do the researchers hope to find out from this trial?*

*What are the possible advantages and risks of taking part?*

*Is the trial randomized?*

*What will I have to do if I join the trial, including tests and check-ups?*

*Can I have tests and treatment at my usual treatment center or will I have to travel?*

*Is there any help available to cover costs?*

*Will joining a trial mean that there are any medicines or treatments I can't have?*

*Is the trial insured?*

*Will taking part in a trial affect my medical insurance?*

## Finding further information and support

It can be difficult to cope when you have an advanced cancer. But you don't have to do it all alone. There may be times when you need the support of others. There are some steps you can take to try to make sure you have all the support you need.

### Find out about NSCLC and its treatment

People vary in how much they want to know when they have a life-threatening illness. Some people want to know everything, while others want to hear as little as possible about their illness or treatment. It's completely up to you.

Being informed about your condition may help you to deal with it. It may give you back a sense of control. The more you know about a situation, the less scary it may seem. And, by being better placed to make decisions about your own treatment, you will be more in control.

You may also get more out of your consultations with your doctors and nurses. If you understand your condition and treatment, it may help you to communicate most effectively with them. And do ask for more explanation if there's anything that's not clear to you.

### Share with your family and friends

It's often said that people don't know what to say when someone close to them has cancer. That can be true. But most people are willing to talk about it – or better still, listen. They may not know whether you want to talk and are waiting for you to bring it up.

Of course, it's entirely your choice who you tell and what you tell them. But sharing what you know and how you feel with your family and friends may help them to cope and to better support you. Tell them you don't expect them to have answers, but that it helps to have someone to listen if you're coming to an important decision.

## Find others in a similar situation

Finding others in a similar situation to you can be an important source of psychological support. Your specialist nurse may know of local support or patient advocacy groups that you can go to.

Local face-to-face support groups are usually for people with all types of cancer so you may not find people in exactly the same situation, but there are likely to be other people who've been told they have an advanced cancer, so they'll have some idea of what it's been like for you.

With online forums, finding other people with the same condition as you is easier than it used to be. A lot of people prefer to make contact online because it's anonymous and can feel safe – you're not so exposed. There are some details at the back of this booklet about support organizations you may find helpful.

## Second opinions

As we've said, your own specialist is best placed to advise you on treatment because they know you so well. However, it's understandable to want to check that what you've been told about your situation is correct.

Most cancer specialists are used to people asking for a second opinion. They understand that you are not questioning their judgement but want to explore every avenue.

If you feel awkward asking your current specialist, you can ask your primary care (general) practitioner. If you are making a private approach to a cancer specialist, you may be able to make an appointment yourself. But it's best to involve your specialist if you can. They will let the doctor providing the second opinion have access to all your scans and test results. If this isn't possible, you may need to have some repeated.

# Guide to words and phrases

**Adenocarcinoma:** A cancer that starts in glandular tissue. A lung adenocarcinoma is a cancer of the gland cells lining the airways.

**Advanced cancer:** Also known as 'metastatic cancer'. Usually means a cancer that has spread from where it started to another part of the body.

**ALK:** A gene that is normally only active during development inside the womb. ALK can fuse with another gene to create a driver mutation in lung cancer cells. It is now used as a target for treatment.

**Amino acid:** A fundamental molecule that, when in a chain with other amino acids, forms a protein.

**Biomarker:** A substance or gene that occurs naturally in the body that can be measured in a medical test. Depending on the substance and the test, a biomarker can measure a normal body process, show that a disease is present, or indicate how a disease is responding to treatment.

**Cancer stage:** A way of classifying cancers by size and whether they have spread. Usually, stages go from 1 to 4, with a stage 1 cancer being localized and a stage 4 cancer having spread to another part of the body.

**Clinical trial:** A carefully designed research study to investigate a new test, treatment, or medical procedure in people.

**DNA:** DNA is the 'blueprint' for life as it controls the growth and function of cells. Genes are made of DNA, and they carry all the instructions for an organism to grow, survive, and reproduce. Each gene carries the instructions to make a single type of protein.

**DNA repair gene:** A gene that codes for one of the key proteins involved in repairing DNA. A mutation in one of these genes can contribute to the development of a cancer.

**Driver mutations:** Abnormal changes in genes that encourage cancer growth, these are the most important mutations in the development of a cancer. Driver mutations can be used by researchers as potential targets for treatment.

**EGFR:** A gene that normally encourages cells to divide. Mutations in EGFR can act as driver mutations in NSCLCs and bowel cancers and are now used as targets for treatment.

**Eligibility criteria:** The set of requirements that govern entry into a clinical trial.

**G12C:** The most common mutation found in the KRAS gene in NSCLCs. It is a driver mutation and now used as a target for treatment.

**Gene:** A unit of DNA that carries the code for a single protein.

**Immune checkpoint inhibitors:** Treatments that prevent cancers from sending signals that switch off the immune system.

**Locally advanced cancer:** The cancer has grown outside the organ that it started in and into surrounding body tissues.

**KRAS:** A gene that is often mutated in NSCLCs. Driver mutations in KRAS encourage cancer cell growth. KRAS is an important predictive biomarker for NSCLC and some other cancers and is now used as a target for treatment.

**Metastasis/metastatic cancer:** A technical term for cancer spreading to another part of the body or body organ. Also known as 'advanced cancer'.

**Monoclonal antibody:** An antibody is an immune system protein. A monoclonal antibody is a single type of antibody that is made in large quantities in a laboratory and used as a medical treatment.

**Mutation:** An abnormality in a gene.

**NSCLC:** Abbreviation for non-small cell lung cancer.

**Oncogene:** Means 'cancer gene'. A normal gene with a mutation that may cause a cell to become a cancer cell and multiply in the body.

**Patient information sheet:** Pages of information that a doctor or researcher must give you before you agree to join a clinical trial. Contains all the important information about the trial, including its aims, the treatment groups, and side effects.

**Phase:** Part of the process a clinical trial. Phase I trials generally look at safety. Phase II trials find out more about side effects and how well treatments work. Phase III trials are the largest and usually randomized. They test potential new treatments against standard treatment to see which works better. Phase IV trials take place after a treatment has been approved.

**Primary cancer:** Where a cancer starts in the body.

**Protein:** The building blocks of the body. Proteins can also act as messages within and between cells, controlling growth and other cellular processes.

**Secondary cancer:** Also called metastatic cancer, a secondary cancer is a tumor in the part of the body a cancer has spread to. If you have an NSCLC that has spread to the liver, you have a primary lung cancer and secondary lung cancer in your liver.

**Systemic therapy:** A treatment that circulates throughout the body. All types of drug treatment are systemic therapies. Surgery and radiotherapy are local therapies as they only treat one part of the body.

**Targeted therapy/treatment:** Cancer treatments that 'target' abnormal proteins made by cancer cells. These abnormal proteins often help tumors grow and spread in the body, so by targeting them, doctors hope to control the cancer.

**Tumor suppressor gene:** A gene that normally switches off cell division and promotes the death of damaged or aging cells. An abnormal tumor suppressor gene will not be able to prevent cancer cells from multiplying.

**Vaccine:** A vaccine is something that stimulates the immune system to produce antibodies to protect against a disease. A cancer vaccine is a type of immunotherapy that helps the body's immune system to fight the cancer.

## Useful resources

**American Cancer Society**
www.cancer.org

**Cancer Research UK database of UK cancer trials**
www.cancerresearchuk.org/about-cancer/find-a-clinical-trial

**European Organisation for the Research and Treatment of Cancer database of European cancer trials**
www.eortc.org/clinical-trials-database

**KRAS Kickers – online support forum for anyone affected by KRAS-positive non-small cell lung cancer**
www.kraskickers.org

**Lung Cancer Europe**
www.lungcancereurope.eu

**Lung Cancer Foundation of America**
https://lcfamerica.org

**Lungevity**
www.lungevity.org

**National Comprehensive Cancer Network – US organization that produces guidelines for patients on cancers, treatments, and side effects**
www.nccn.org/patientresources/patient-resources/guidelines-for-patients

**US National Library of Medicine database of clinical trials**
https://clinicaltrials.gov

## Sources used in the preparation of this document

**American Cancer Society**
www.cancer.org

**American Society of Clinical Oncology**
www.cancer.net

**Cancer Research UK**
www.cancerresearchuk.org

**Lung Cancer Foundation of America**
https://lcfamerica.org

**Lungevity**
www.lungevity.org

**Medline Plus**
https://medlineplus.gov

**National Cancer Institute**
www.cancer.gov

Fast Facts for Patients

Oncology — Pneumology


**Contributors**

**Dr Anne-Marie Baird**, Trinity College Dublin and Lung Cancer Europe

**Dr Hossein Borghaei**, Fox Chase Cancer Center

**Terri Conneran**, KRAS Kickers

**Dr Devika Das**, University of Alabama at Birmingham

**Dr Ticiana Leal**, Winship Cancer Institute, Emory University

**Dr Howard (Jack) West**, City of Hope Comprehensive Cancer Center



Medical writing support provided by Liz Woolf.

Although this booklet has been supported with funding from Mirati Therapeutics, Inc., the opinions expressed are those of the writer and contributors.





ISBN: 978-3-318-07249-5


**We'd like your feedback**

How has this booklet helped you? Is there anything you didn't understand? Do you still have any unanswered questions?

Please send your questions, or any other comments, to fastfacts@karger.com and help readers of future editions. Thank you!

Karger

HEALTHCARE